THE AIDS DONOR

Marquiessa Monique Rhodes

Copyright © 2009 by Marquiessa Monique Rhodes

All rights reserved.

No part of this publication may be reproduced, distributed, or transmitted in any form or by any means, including photocopying, recording, or other electronic or mechanical methods, without the prior written permission of the publisher, except as permitted by U.S. copyright law. For permission requests, contact Rhodeo Enterprise by email at rhodeoenterprise@gmail.com.

The story, all names, characters, and incidents portrayed in this production are fictitious. No identification with actual persons (living or deceased), places, buildings, and products is intended or should be inferred.

First US edition 2024

TABLE OF CONTENTS

This book is dedicated to Gerard Nero for being a friend, an inspiration and a motivator. This book wouldn't be published without you.

INTRODUCTION

It's funny how when we are kids we listen to things that we think are harmless, we see things that we think are harmless, but little do we know that those things actually do affect us when we get older. I remember hearing about AIDs and HIV back in the late 80s when it first came on the scene. I was never really scared of it because I looked at it as a gay man's disease. At least that's what it seemed like it was because all you saw were gay men getting it.

Then in the 90s, the rapper Easy-E caught it and died from it. I think that scared people because with him dying, now we knew that it was more than just a gay man's disease. Magic Johnson said that he had it. But then he didn't die like everyone else that had it. He kept living and looking healthy and because of that, going into the early 2000s, AIDs/HIV was no longer scary to people. Well, it was no longer scary to me. All these new drugs were introduced to slow the virus down. This just meant that people wouldn't look like they had AIDs/HIV anymore.

The infected ones would be hard to identify. So what did we have to fear? I mean, if Magic could live forever with it then why would I be scared to get it? As a society, we haven't done enough to prevent AIDs/HIV from happening. There are so many kids out there that will grow up with a mindset just like me. I was careless. I went through life thinking that I could identify the disease by looking at people. I was wrong.

But no one taught me so that I could understand. My Parents? My parents tried to hide the truth about sex from me, afraid that they may influence me to have sex. What they failed to realize is that when they didn't tell me everything, I mean everything, they influenced me to want to have sex. In school, they taught us to be abstinent. They didn't teach us about STDs, the signs and symptoms or the importance of wearing a condom. They just told us not to have sex.

What kid you know in the 20st century that wants to hear about abstinence? Not this one. But I needed them to teach me about protecting myself and getting tested. Maybe put it on TV or on the radio.

I needed to see people reaching for condoms before they were about to have sex. Instead I saw them in the movies or on television, just going at it. That's what I saw, so that is what I tried to mimic.

Sex seemed to me as the best and most important thing in this world. I knew that when I got old enough, I had to get it. And I did. Lots of it. I abused sex. I ignored all the bad sides to it, and the deadly consequences. I just wanted to have a good time. I just wanted lots of women. And I got both. And then I got AIDs too. Now I am worried that every kid in America will end up just like me; infected with the AIDs virus and spreading it to more people. That's not what I want for the kids in America. I want them to be informed. That is why I have to tell them my story. I have got to tell them how I became the AIDs Donor!

Quincy Carter

CHAPTER 1

The Infamous Quincy Carter

"We are on the record. It's the state of Georgia versus Quincy Carter!" said Judge Matthews, the judiciary presiding over the AIDs murder case.

"Is the prosecution ready to call its first witness?"

"Yes, we are your honor!" said Brad Adams, the leading attorney for the prosecution. "The state calls Ms. Shirley James."

Shirley got up from the pit wearing a pink sun dress and walked to the stand. She then raised her hand and swore to tell the truth, the whole truth and nothing but the truth.

"State your name for the jury please." asked Mr. Adams.

"Shirley James!" she responded.

"Ms. James, do you know the defendant?"

"Yes, I do!" answered Shirley.

"And how do you know him?" asked Mr. Adams.

"I met him one night at a hitting club in Atlanta. He was there with a couple of his boys.

They were all looking good and dressed well, but Quincy stood out the most. He was clean from head to toe. His hair was nicely cut, his clothes were fresh, his teeth were clean and straight and his smile lit up the room.

He just had this professional, confident look about him. He was quite a catch. I spotted him while on the dance floor with a few of my girlfriends. Our eyes met and then he came over to me, gently put his arms around my waist and whispered

"hey baby!" in my ear. It was such a turn on, that he had me from there."

"So does that mean you went home and slept with him that night?" asked Mr. Adams.

"No, we just exchanged numbers." Shirley responded.
"Okay. Let's fast forward to the night that you did sleep with him. Tell me what happened that night." demanded the attorney.

"Well, besides getting a deadly disease, it happened to be one of the best nights of my life. He'd treated me like no other man had. He invited me to his house. It was a penthouse on the top floor of this apartment building downtown.

The place was beautiful. I am talking glass windows everywhere with a view to die for. He had an open floor plan with high ceilings and marble floors. It was everything. In his large kitchen, he'd cooked dinner and set the table with winery and candles. After we ate, we danced, sang songs and had several intimate conversations. It was great. The mood was right and I couldn't help but to sleep with him." she cried and lowered her head into the palms of her hands.

Mr. Adams walked closer and touched her hand.

"You don't have to cry Shirley. It's okay! Now, tell me, before you slept with him, did he attempt to put on a condom?

"No! He damn well didn't even try!" Shirley shouted. "Did he even have the decency to tell you he had a deadly disease?" asked Mr. Adams.

"No, he didn't. And you would think a man of his caliber wouldn't do such a thing." said Shirley.

"What do you mean by a man of his caliber? What kind of person is he?"

"You would never expect a man like him to have AIDs, HIV or any other sexually transmitted disease. He seemed too intelligent, too educated, too professional, too well put together for that to happen to him. I mean look at him," Shirley pointed at Quincy, "does he look like someone that would have HIV?"

"But he did have it, and now so do you. How does that make you feel Ms. James?"

"I really can't explain how I felt. Words just can't explain those feelings.

I was so depressed, hurt and shameful, while at the same time very angry.

I wanted to die more than anything. I have kids. How am I supposed to tell them that one day soon mommy is going to die from an STD?

How can I look them in their eyes and tell them that I am dying from the AIDs virus?"

 Shirley broke down in tears once again.

"Ms. James, one more question. What do you think should happen to Mr. Carter?"

Shirley yelled, "He needs to be killed or locked away somewhere and tortured every day of his life.
A man like him, doesn't deserve to live!"

"Thank you Ms. James. No further questions your honor." said Mr. Adams.

"Mr. Jackson, your witness!" said Judge Matthews.

Mr. Jackson, the defense attorney for Quincy Carter, stood up and approached the stand.

"Ms. James, when things got heated at Mr. Carter's home, did you stop to ask him to put on a condom?"

"No, I did not!" Shirley firmly stated as if she could not believe he was asking her that question.

"Why not?" asked Mr. Jackson.

"Because I got caught up in the moment and at the time a condom was not on my mind.

That's never happened to you before?" asked Shirley.

"Ms. James I am not the one on trial right now." Mr. Jackson laughed along with the rest of the court.

"Let me get this straight, you didn't ask him to use a condom because you got caught up in the moment, is that correct?"

"Yes, that's correct!"

"Ms. James are you aware that there are millions of people infected with HIV/AIDs in the United States?" asked Mr. Jackson.

"Well, I knew the virus was out there, but I did not know that it affected that many people. I thought maybe it was like a few thousands a year." said Shirley unsure of her answer.

"Even knowing that there are thousands of cases every year, why wouldn't you at least try to protect yourself from any disease? Are you telling me that you were too caught up in the moment to think about your own personal safety?"

"I guess!" said Shirley getting irritated with Mr. Jackson's questions.

"You guess? Ms. James have you had unprotected sex before?"

"Yes, I have!" Shirley whispered.

"About how many times would you say that you have? Give me a percentage. 50% of the time, 90% of the time, how often Ms. James?"

"Not all the time. Only half of the time and most of that time is when I think I can trust that person." said Shirley.

"Ms. James do you not know that over half of the people infected with this disease don't even know they are infected and you are trusting them to know? And to add to that, you are telling me that half of the time that you are sexually active, you are welcoming diseases to just come in and reside in your body?!"

"OBJECTION, YOUR HONOR!" screamed Mr. Adams.
"OVERRULED!" said Judge Matthews.

"Ms. James please answer the question."
"I don't welcome diseases." Shirley responded.

"Ms. James you are having unprotected sex half of the time you have sex which means you are welcoming diseases into your body. Have you had a disease before Ms. James?"
"Yes!" she answered softly.

"What was that Ms. James? Can you say it a little louder so the rest of the court can hear you?!" asked Mr. Jackson.

"I said, yes!" Shirley screamed. "I've had Chlamydia before, once."

"So even after getting one disease, you didn't learn your lesson. You didn't attempt to prevent it from happening a second time. Now look what happened. You got something even worse than Chlamydia. You got a deadly disease."

"OBJECTION, YOUR HONOR. WHO IS ON TRIAL HERE?" Mr. Adams jumped up.

"SUSTAINED. MR. JACKSON DO NOT BADGER THE WITNESS." stated Judge Matthews.
"One last question, your honor." said Mr. Jackson.

"Ms. James, if you couldn't protect yourself from getting a disease, why should we feel sorry for you because you got the AIDs virus from unprotected sex?"

"Because I didn't ask for this disease! He knew what he was doing before he even slept with me. He deserves to rot in hell. I have to pay for what he has done?

Other women have to pay too? You should be ashamed of yourself for defending him. What kind of man are you? Obviously one that doesn't have a daughter. You let him go then you are letting all the HIV predators go! I guess its ok for people to go around giving out a deadly disease. I hope he gets the electric chair!"

"Thank you Ms. James!" said Mr. Jackson.

"The death penalty!" screamed Ms. James
"Thank you Ms. James! No further questions your honor." Ms. James quickly got up and went back to her seat. Mr.

Adams then called his next witness, Kesha Collins.
"Ms. Collins, how are you today?" asked Mr. Adams.
"Fine, thank you!" replied Kesha.

"Ms. Collins, can you identify for the court the man that gave you the AIDs virus?" asked attorney Adams.

Kesha pointed directly at Quincy and said, "Yes, I can. He's right there, Quincy. The guy in the nice blue suit"

"Kesha, how did you meet Quincy?"

"I met him in the mall one day. He was in Foot Locker buying some sneaks.

I was in there buying my nephew some basketball shoes. Somehow we ended up looking in the same shoe section. He made a few jokes, I laughed and then he introduced himself. He told me he was new in town and then he asked me if I could show him around. I said yes and asked him where he would like to go. He said he would like to take me to a nice restaurant of my choice. Of course I said yes. This was my opportunity to go to a very nice, upscale restaurant at someone else's expense," she laughed.

"So you went to dinner with him? What happened after dinner? Did you sleep with him?" asked Mr. Adams. "We went back to his place and watched a horror flick." said Kesha.

"Did you sleep with him?"
"Yes, unfortunately for me, I did!"
"Did anything he did or say lead you to believe that he a had disease?" asked Mr. Adams.

"No, I never suspected he had a disease and he never said anything about having a disease either," replied Kesha.

"So how did you feel once you found out you'd been infected?"

"I just busted into tears. Then I got angry. I wanted to kill him. I tried contacting him to confront him about what he'd done, but he wouldn't answer his phone or his door. It made me even madder. I just wanted to kill him!

"You mean to tell me he avoided you after he knew he'd infected you? What kind of a man does such a thing?" He turned to the audience. "I'll tell you what kind of a man does such a thing. A sick man, an inconsiderate man! A selfish man, and downright no good man! That man, everybody is Quincy Carter!" said the attorney as he walked back to his seat.

Mr. Jackson stood up and started his questioning.

"Ms. Collins, you stated earlier that you slept with Quincy on the first night. Correct?"

"Yes, I slept with him on the first night but if you are implying that it was like a one night stand, then no, it was nothing like that."

"And the night you had sex with him, didn't he attempt to put on a condom? Wasn't it your bright idea for him to take the condom off?"

"Yes, but you don't understand my reasons for doing so." said Kesha on the defensive.

"What's your reason, Ms. Collins? What could possibly prevent you from wearing a condom besides the fact that you just simply didn't want to?"

"Yes, he did put on a condom!" shouted Kesha over the noise from the audience.

The audience couldn't believe what they were hearing.

"Secondly, I only asked him to remove it because I am allergic to latex condoms. With that said it is still his responsibility to tell me if he had something or not."

"Allergic to latex condoms?!" he smiled.

"Come on Ms. Collins, you can do better than that. Let me give some facts. Fact #1, there are condoms out there that are non-latex condoms. Fact #2, there are also female condoms out there just in case your boyfriend or lover forgets his.

You know the more I hear these stories, the less I feel sorry for you and the rest of these women. You all put yourselves at risk and now you want to use my client as an excuse as to why you all were irresponsible for your own health. I've heard enough." said a disgusted Mr. Jackson.

As he turned his back to walk away, Kesha stood up and shouted at him,

"Wait a minute, Mr. Jackson. How dare you speak to me in such a way? You don't know what I've been through." she cried.

"When I was a young lady, and I was sexually active, I tried to get boys to wear a condom, but none of them liked it.

Every time I pushed for us to be safe, they pushed against it. They said the sex felt better without condoms. Then they would assure me that they cared about me and wouldn't hurt me, so I believed them. I didn't want to lose any of my boyfriends so I did what I needed to please them. I just wanted to be liked or loved. I just wanted them to desire me. I wanted to make them happy and if that meant not wearing a condom, then that's what I did.

I grew up believing that God put us on this Earth to procreate so as a woman you should always have a man, and to get a one, sometimes that meant bending the rules." she continued crying.

Mr. Jackson turned around and handed her his hanky and then continued to his seat. He'd heard enough for the day.

CHAPTER 2

The Trial

"The prosecution calls Ms. Lauren Phillips," said attorney Adams.

"Ms. Phillips, please state your name for the jury."

"Lauren Shanee' Phillips."

"Ms. Phillips, how did you meet Mr. Carter?"

"I've known Quincy for years. We grew up together. I've known him for over 10 years."

"And how long have you been sleeping with him?"

"Over 5 years now."

"And how long have you been sleeping with him unprotected?"

"Ummm....five years on and off!" she smiled.

"And has Quincy been the only one for the past 5 years?"

"No!"

"So it's safe to say that my client may not for sure be the one that infected you?"

"No, I know Quincy gave me this disease. He is the only man I would sleep with without a condom."

"And why is that?"

"Because I've known him all my life. I trusted him. I would never expect Quincy to have anything. You think it's easy to tell someone you've been with for years to wear a condom?

It's not. They easily get offended and think that you don't trust them. You know I am kind of disappointed in him because I thought he cared more about me. I still can't believe he has done this to me. He really hurt me." "When you discovered that you'd been infected, was it easy for you to get in contact with him?"

"No, it wasn't. He wouldn't answer the phone and he was nowhere to be found. I think it's because he felt really bad for what he did. Of all the women here, I don't think he wanted to infect me."

"How did you feel when you found out?"

"For a long time I lived in isolation. I didn't want to see nobody. Then, I felt like killing someone; him in particular.

I rode by his house several times, waiting for him to show up so I could shoot him in the back.

I hated him and I hated myself. I really don't want to live anymore and nor do I want him to live either. "Should Mr. Carter go to jail for what he's done?"

"No, he needs to be killed and if the jury won't do it, I will." "Thank you Ms. Phillips." said Mr. Adams. "No further questions your honor."

Mr. Jackson stood up and began questioning Ms. Phillips. "Ms. Phillips, you stated that you would be healthy had it not been for the disease my client gave you?"

"Yes, that's correct!"

"You slept with my client over the past 5 years, if I recall correctly?"

"Yes!"

"How long have you had the virus?"

"I would say about the same amount of time."

"The same amount of time? Are you sure about that Ms. Phillips?

Because from the looks of your medical records," he went to the desk and picked up Lauren's records,

" You've been infected with the HIV for over seven years, which means you gave my client HIV and he gave it to these women.
If this is true, Ms. Phillips, then you should be the one on trial here and not my client."

"What! He gave me this disease and he gave those women HIV! Do not try to turn this case on me Mr. Jackson. Your client had HIV! He didn't get it from me. He deserves to be on trial and he deserves everything that is coming to him."

"Ms. Phillips, I have spoken with old co-workers and they tell me that years ago you were very sick.

They say you were passing out at work, having hot spells, and that you also had lesions on your face. Is this true,

Ms. Phillips?"
"I was sick, but that doesn't mean I had HIV. People have hot spells when they have a fever. People pass out when they aren't hydrated, and they get pimples and bumps on their face all the time. That man right there, Quincy Carter, gave me this disease."

"Well, it's hard for me to believe that my client gave you that disease when you already had it over 7 years ago. No further questions your honor," attorney Jackson said as he took his seat.

The court was ordered to take a fifteen minute recess. During the recess attorney Jackson met with the last crucial witness of the day, Crystal Jones. They talked and went over a few questions. While talking to Crystal the other ladies approached Attorney Jackson with a few questions of their own.

"What the hell is going on Jack?" asked Kesha.

The other ladies looked in as if they wanted to ask the same question.

"You are making us look stupid up there. We agreed to this little plan of Quincy's but we are the ones looking bad here. If I am not mistaken, I would say Quincy is trying to betray us. Are you guys trying to betray us Jack?"

"Calm down ladies. Nobody is being betrayed here.

Everything that is happening is routine," said Jack. "Routine, huh, Jack?

Looks to me as if you are trying to win this case, and that was not part of the plan," said Kesha.

"Quincy will do what he promised, if you ladies do what you promised. So far you have not fulfilled your end of the bargain. You betrayed Quincy first and I am not going to sit here and let him go down by himself," said attorney Jackson. Crystal was confused and curious at the same time to know what was going on.

"What's going on here?" interrupted Crystal. "What are you guys talking about? What plan?" "Nothing!" said Jack.

"Well, it sounds like something to me. I want to know what it is or I am not taking that stand? Tell me now or I will turn and walk away. Jack?!" demanded Crystal.

"Hhhhhuuuu...!" sighed Jack.

He looked at all the ladies for confirmation. As soon as he started to talk, the fifteen minute recess had expired.

"Whew....looks like I will have to tell you when we have time. But for now, can I count on you to testify?" he asked. "Ms. Jones?! Ms. Jones?! Will you take the stand?"

"I will take the stand if you promise to tell me what's going on."

"I promise to tell you after we finish the court session today. You have my word."

Jack made his promise and then they returned to the courtroom.

"Your honor the defense calls Ms. Crystal Jones," said Mr. Jackson.

Crystal took the stand, put her left hand on the bible, raised her right hand and swore to tell the truth and nothing but the truth.

"Ms. Jones, how did you meet Mr. Carter?"
"I met him at a basketball game and we hit it off from there."
"Did you sleep with him?"
"Yes, I slept with him!"
"And are you infected with the AIDs virus, Ms. Jones?"
"No!"

The crowded Ooooed. They could not believe it. How could this woman have slept with an HIV infected man and not have the disease? Crystal was one of the 3 women that was not infected by Quincy that actually testified.

"Ms. Jones, could you please explain to the court the reason why you were not infected by Mr. Carter?" asked attorney Jackson.

"Because I protected myself. I used a condom, that was the only way I was going to sleep with him. No condom, no ass!" "You used a condom?!" smiled attorney Jackson as he turned to the audience.

 "So let me get this straight Ms. Jones, you asked Mr. Carter to put on a condom and he did? And because he did, you did not get infected?"

"Yes, that is correct. He seemed to have no problem wearing a condom."

"Magically, somehow the three women that did ask him to wear a condom do not have the disease, but the ten women that refused to wear the condoms do.

Do you have any idea as to how this could have happened?

I mean do you think wearing a condom played a big part in that or do you think the three of you were just lucky and they weren't. Please explain it to the jury for me if you can."

"Of course wearing a condom played a big part in it. I am glad I have always been the type of woman that will not engage in any sexual act without protecting myself.

Had I said no to that condom at least once, just once then I would probably be an AIDs victim also. So I am very happy that I wore that condom," Crystal smiled.

"Do you think Quincy should die or go to jail for what he did?

"No, I don't think he should go to jail or die. Quincy is not responsible for what has happened to these women. What happened to these women was preventable and they chose not to prevent it from happening. We are talking about grown women here. They should be responsible for their own lives. Should Quincy go to jail? No, because that won't help the HIV problems of today, that will just make it worse.

I think he should be out in the community servicing our country. He should be out there educating the young sexually active, illiterate kids. They need to make that his community service. We need someone, well someone that is infected, to go out into the community and tell their story so these kids won't think that everything about sex is a good thing."

"Thank you Crystal. No further questions your honor."

Mr. Jackson smiled at Attorney Adams as he went back to his seat. Attorney Adams then stood up and began questioning Ms. Jones.

"Ms. Jones, were you upset to hear that Quincy had slept with you when he knowingly had a disease?" asked Attorney Adams.

"Yes and no!" answered Crystal.

"Yes and no? Please elaborate for the jury Ms. Jones."

"Yes because I keep wondering what if the condom had busted or somehow came off. I would be screwed. I would be infected too. I am upset with myself for not making him get tested, but I am also proud of myself for practicing safe sex. I love myself way too much to take such crazy risks.

Apparently these women do not love themselves enough to let it happen to them. No man means that much to me to make me do harm to myself. Never! A man does not love you if he cannot protect you; sexually that is."

"Ms. Jones, you say Quincy shouldn't go to jail for what he's done? Maybe you say that because you aren't infected, but what if you were infected would your answer be different?" asked the attorney.

"I don't know!"
Crystal responded.

"Let's go back to the night you slept with him. What if the condom he was wearing popped and you did get infected, how do you think you would feel?"

"Terrible, I guess. I would probably feel like the rest of these women. But I really can't say how I would feel because I did not get infected."

"Thank you Ms. Jones! No further questions your honor." And that was it for that day. They only had one day of trial remaining. Quincy would be the last and only witness left to testify.

As everyone exited the court, Crystal made it her business to ensure that Jack didn't get away from telling her about this plan.

"Okay, Jack, you gave me your word so spill it!" she demanded.

"Sure, but not here. Come and take a ride with me and we will talk about it." Jack insisted.

Crystal agreed. They walked out of the court room and into the parking lot. They then took a ride in Jack's convertible Mustang.

"You feel like hearing a long story?" asked Jack.

"Sure, as long as it's about the plan," answered Crystal. "Oh, It is! It is! Just sit back and relax. This is going to be a long story."

CHAPTER 3

The Plan

"It had been a long year for Quincy. He'd graduated from a prestigious University in North Carolina and landed a job at one of the top Investment firms in Atlanta, Georgia. This would be his first time away from home. Atlanta was something new to him. The women were everywhere. He had no problem finding places to meet women and if he did, he just went to the strip club and paid for sex.

Every weekend he would take a different woman home and have sex with her. He would pick and choose which ones he wanted to use a condom with and which ones he wanted to do unprotected. He figured the prettiest and sexiest girls would be the disease free ones because they were just too fine to die, and the not so pretty ones would be the ones to use the condom with because they just didn't look right. Quincy went nine months with the same routine until one day he noticed something different about his health. He was often feeling nauseated, faint and dizzy.

He was occasionally sweating in his sleep for no reason. He had hot flashes and sometimes weird marks would appear on his body. He didn't know what was going on but he knew he couldn't ignore it so he scheduled a doctor's appointment for a regular checkup. He tested for diabetes, and high blood pressure but every test he took came up negative. Something was wrong with him but he figured he would give it a week to clear up, and if it didn't clear up, he would get tested for STDs.

Quincy waited a week and all that week he'd felt the same. He really didn't want to get tested. He didn't want anyone to see him going to the clinic. He was scared that he would run into someone and they would think he already had something. He had convinced himself that if he did have a disease he didn't want to know anything about it. He would be too embarrassed if he did. He couldn't hold out for long though, the symptoms were getting out of control. He had to know what was going on with him so he could fix it. So he just accepted the consequences and went to the local clinic where it was free for STD testing.

That day in the lobby as he waited to be called, he realized that he may have been wrong about STDs. He saw all kinds of people at the clinic, blacks, Mexicans, whites, thugs, pretty girls, ugly girls, old people and young people. There wasn't just one type of person in there as he suspected; it was all types of persons. This made him kind nervous because he knew then that he was not special and could possibly have a disease. After an hour of sitting and waiting Quincy's name was finally called. He got up and went to the back for testing. After a week had passed, he received his test results back for

Chlamydia, Gonorrhea, Herpes, and Syphilis.

His results stated that he was negative. Quincy was in high spirits. He just knew he was good. Well, that was, until his HIV results arrived. In exactly 16 days, the clinic called Quincy to come in. Quince waited a couple of days before he would show. He was too afraid of the results. After two days, he'd waited long enough. The time for him to get the results were overdue, so he went in. Waiting in the lobby once again, he could feel the pressure building up. His heart was beating faster than normal.

Sweat dripped from his face and his legs were shaking out of control. Finally they'd called him to the back room. He got up and walked towards the room. He entered the room and was asked to take a seat. The counselor asked him a few questions. They asked him if he was sexually active, and if he gave or received oral sex, or both. You know, the usual questioning when you go for checkup."

Crystal shook her head as a way of saying she understood what he was talking about.

"Well, Quincy answered yes to almost all the questions. After that the doctor gave Quincy the bad news. Quincy had tested positive for the Human Immune Deficiency Virus.

Quincy was stunned. He just couldn't believe he was HIV positive.

He went home and trashed his place out of anger. He destroyed everything in his house until there was nothing left to destroy. At this point, he'd exhausted himself, making it a perfect time for him to sit and reflect on what just happened to him. He reassessed the situation and convinced himself that maybe the test was inaccurate. So he took another test.

That one came up positive.

He took another one. Over the next two months he'd taken at least five tests and every last one of them came up with the same result, positive. He was no longer in denial, and he was no longer a happy man."

Crystal was enjoying the story but she didn't know what it had to do with The Plan.

"What does this have to do with The Plan Jack? Tell me about The Plan." she demanded.

"I am getting to the plan, Crystal. Please be patient. You must know why there is a plan first before you know what the plan is. Now with that said, may I continue my story?"

"Yes," answered Crystal.

"Quincy had finally accepted the fact that he had the disease. He no longer wanted to be around people anymore. He quit his job and for months he laid in his bed depressed, wishing for that unlucky day to come. He would go weeks without showering. He barely paid his bills. For the life of him he just couldn't believe he had HIV. Because he was rich and attractive, he thought he didn't fit the criteria.

One depressing day, laid out on the couch, he read an article about the rise of HIV/AIDS in the black community in an edition of the Essence Magazine. There were articles and articles on beautiful people that had been infected with the disease. And like Quincy, each person had experienced moods of depression and also had suicidal tendencies. But these people had found a way to turn their lives around by being a voice in their communities.

The article touched Quincy so deeply that he wanted to do his part in the community. He quickly became a spokesman for HIV awareness and prevention. His first experience was speaking to teenagers but it wasn't easy. Most of them didn't care much for abstinence or sex education so Quincy did the best he could.

He talked about the different types of people that could get it, the different types of diseases, how to prevent and how to treat each disease. He even talked about the number of infected African Americans. And although he was well prepared and his presentations were outstanding, he didn't feel as though his message was getting through to the kids.

They kept finding reasons to believe the disease couldn't be as serious as he suggested.   As much as he tried, he could not convince them. It was a lost cause. He became frustrated.

He knew he couldn't get through to the kids by his words only. He knew he had to show them, rather than just tell them. So that's when he decided to sleep around."

"Oh my God!" said Crystal. "He did all of this to prove a point to some kids?"

"He needed to find a way to show the importance of contraception and also the severity of HIV/AIDs in the community. One day he called me and asked me to come over to his house. There he told me his life story and why he felt as though he needed to do something to slow this AIDs thing down in the community. I think his childhood is much like most of the kids that grow up in lower income families.

When he was young, he grew up watching pornos, thinking that was the way sex was supposed to be. And on those pornos he never saw anyone wearing condoms. I mean today they wear condoms in pornos, but back in the day, they never did. You know what he told me?" asked Jack.

"What's that?" asked Crystal.

"He said his first cassette tape was a single by the rapper J-Dub called "Hit it Raw""

Jack laughed. "I went out and bought the cd to see what Quincy was talking about.

Would you like to hear the song?"

Crystal nodded her head as Jack looked for the disc. Finally he'd located the disc in his glove compartment. He put the disc in and the lyrics played:

All I got is you,

And all you got is me

So girl let's get together

So you can get the "d"

Don't worry about the condom

Cause we can take the flaw

It just feels damn good when

you let me hit it raw

Hit it raw...Hey...Hit it raw(ain't got no time to put no condom on).

Hit it raw....Hey ...Hit it raw(cause that would just take too long)

Hit it raw...Hey....Hit it raw(girl all i want to do is bone)
Hit it raw,....Hey...Hit it raw(just get on me and get your grind on) They both laughed.

"That's crazy, isn't it? Poor guy. He couldn't help but to grow up sexually illiterate."

"Yeah, it is sad!" answered Crystal.

"Quincy was convinced that the kids from low income families, trailer parks, and the ghettos would never be fully educated on Sexually Transmitted Diseases and how to prevent them. He wanted to teach them how to protect themselves from these diseases.

He wanted to show them the consequences of having unprotected sex but he just did not know how to do it. The day he'd called me over to his house, he'd come up with a plan. He wanted to see how many women he could sleep with and infect without contraception. He wanted to see how many of them would easily trust him because of his appearance and he wanted to see how many of them would get tested.

He planned to sleep with 15 women and after he'd slept with the last one, he would call all of them and tell them that he had the disease. Then he would offer to pay for their medication and go to jail in exchange for their testimony. But in these testimonies, he wanted these women to take responsibility for their own actions. He wanted them to say that they were part of the reasons as to why they have the disease because they didn't use protection. If they agreed to do that, then he agreed to show up in court and purposely lose the case."

"What?!" asked Crystal. "Why would anyone agree to do that?"

"Because for one, all those women did not even know they were infected. Secondly, Quincy is willing to take responsibility for what he has done. How many people you know that are willing to call all the people they have slept with and tell them they have HIV?" asked Jack.

"Not many," answered Crystal.

"Well Quincy did. And he knew that if he stepped foot in that court, the odds would be against him.

The ladies are getting the good end of the stick. If Quincy loses, he is going to jail and they are going to kill him. He doesn't seem to care about that though. He just wants his message to get across. He just wants the world to see the repercussions of being irresponsible when it comes to not protecting yourself during sex. It's crazy, I know, but it's kind of inspiring."

"So how did he get the ladies to agree to this plan?" asked Crystal.

 "Well after he convinced me to be his attorney, most of the ladies believed he was serious and decided to jump in. And after the others realized they couldn't afford the medication to stay healthy, they agreed to it also. But things aren't going as planned. The ladies are trying to blame everything on Quincy and not themselves.

They are violating our agreement. I can't let them screw Quincy over like that. I plan to win this case for him."

"Wow!" said Crystal, "How do you plan to do that?"
"You will see tomorrow when Quincy testifies."

That was the end of the conversation. Jack dropped Crystal off at her house and took himself home. The next morning he had to prepare for his closing statement.

CHAPTER 4

The Last Drink

It was the final day of the trial and Quincy was the last one to take the stand. The day was long and painful, but somehow his lawyer managed a victory. Based on the irresponsibility of the 10 women, the jury found Quincy not guilty and dropped all charges. The state was enraged. No one could understand the jury's decision, and because of it, Quincy became an everyday target.

He was criticized by the media, by the public and even his own neighbors. Pretty soon he'd become an outcast. He stayed to himself mostly and rarely left the house unless he really needed to. Then one day, months after the trial, he received a phone call from Shirley James.

"Hello?" said Shirley.

"Hi!" answered Quincy.

"Hi, Quince...It's Shirley, Shirley James. Wait! Don't hang up!"

"What do you want Shirley?!"

"I just wanted to call and apologize for the way I treated you in court, and for the way everyone else is treating you. I know it must be hard taking all this criticism from the entire world."

Quincy just listened.

"You know, I never took into consideration that at one point in your life, you'd trusted a woman and she'd infected you. I'm sorry I didn't see that before."

"You are sorry?!" he laughed.

 "Shirley you can't be serious. Aren't you the one that said I should be left somewhere to die? Why should I believe that your apology is sincere?"

"I don't know. I guess because I thought about things and realized that it really wasn't all your fault. I should have looked out for myself. I should have asked you to wear the condom. You would think that a woman my age would know how important that is. I can't blame you for what happened Quincy. It's not your fault. I am the one to blame." she stated.

"Wow, Shirley! I don't know what to say. You really surprised me with that."

As they continued talking, Shirley slowly gained Quincy's trust. For weeks, every day, they would have hour long conversations. Then one day, Shirley broke the ice and asked if they could start seeing each other again. She felt it was a good idea since they were both infected with the virus. Quincy was cautious at first, but after careful thought concluded that it was not a bad idea.

That weekend they had dinner at Quincy's house. They talked, laughed and they drank fabulous wines. Every minute was exciting. Neither of them wanted it to end. Before they knew it the timer on the stove sounded and the entree was ready. Quincy got up and made his way to the kitchen. Before he left the room, he made sure he told Shirley to keep his wine on ice for the next conversation. Little did he know that glass of wine would be his last drink of wine for the night. As he exited the room, Shirley made her move.

She reached into her purse and pulled out two Rhoypnol (Roofies) pills and dropped them into Quincy's wine glass.

When he returned, she greeted him with a smile.

"Hmmm......smells good and looks delicious!" said Shirley. Quincy walked in with a rotisserie chicken.

"Thank you! Now, continue telling me about the time you and your sorority sisters set up that guy in college," he said as he put down the chicken and picked up his wine for a sip.

Shirley continued her story until Quincy was passed out on the floor. She walked over to him and tapped him on the shoulder to make sure he wasn't conscious. Once she was sure that he was out, she ran to the front door and motioned for the other women to come in.

It was nine other women, the divine 9. They had been staking outside of Quincy's house waiting for a signal from Shirley to come in. Things were going as planned. The night of the case, Shirley and a few of the women on the case got together, recruited other women and vowed to find a humiliating way to end Quincy Carter's life.

The ladies entered the home and saw Quincy passed out on the floor. They gathered around him.

"Should we do this while he is asleep or should we wake him up and do it?" asked one girl.

"If we want to torture him, I'd say, let's do it while he is awake," said Shirley.

"Naw. It is better if he doesn't see our faces. It is better if he doesn't know that he is infected with more diseases. We shouldn't tell him, just like he didn't tell us," argued Kesha.

All the women agreed.

"So what's the plan?" asked Shirley.

"The same as before. He will just be asleep. Take his clothes off so we can share these juices with him," Kesha demanded.

The ladies quickly took off Quincy's clothes. They rolled him on his back so his genitals were exposed.

"Well hello there Quincy!" Shirley whispered to his penis. All the women laughed.

"What a waste of a good penis!"

The women shook their heads in agreeance.

"Quincy was always good at pleasing me. I haven't had an orgasm since we stopped sleeping together. I miss him!" said one of the girls.

"Me too!"

"Me too!"

"Me as well!"

Echoed around the room.

"I mean, can't we just forgive him? He is infected. We are infected. We can just be with him, have sex with him and be infected together. Ya'll agree?" asked Shirley. She had convinced most but Kesha wasn't having it.

"Hell no! We are not forgiving him! I wouldn't have this disease if it wasn't for him. It will NEVER go away.

I will have HIV for the rest of my life. I hate him for that. I can't be with men like I used to anymore. I can't love anyone. I can't even kiss on my kids like I want to out of fear of giving them what I have. Quincy has to die! Where is that girl Tina? Get over here!"

Kesha motioned for Tina to come forward.

Tina was an old stripper with Genital Herpes. She had met Quincy a few years ago and wanted to help the ladies out. She walked up and smiled at Quincy.

"I heard you like sharing diseases?" she said as she took off her bottoms to expose her genitals. Then she kneeled down next to the head of his body.

"Well, let me share mine with you."

Down below you could see where she had a break out. She took that area and sat it on Quincy's face.

"Ride his face! Get all up in his mouth!" shouted Kesha. "How long should it take before he has a break out?" ask Kesha.

"A couple of days, maybe weeks." answered Shirley.

"Weeks?!" shouted Lauren. "I want him dead now. Where's that syphilis chick?"

They called for Suzanne, the syphilis chick. She walked up to Quincy's body. The disease was written all over her face.

The room cleared as she got close. No one wanted to be touched by her. She kneeled down and hugged Quincy and then rubbed her face against his. She made her way down to his genital area and started giving him a blow job while at the same time, rubbing her syphilis juices up and down his scrotum. Then she got up and left the room. Her work was done.

The ladies cleaned Quincy up and put his clothes back on. Then they agreed to meet up for the grand finale in about month. Shirley saw them out of the house and then waited for Quincy to gain consciousness again.

After a few hours the drug had worn off and Quincy was awake. When his eyes opened, the first thing he saw was Shirley leaning over him. She was shaking him, asking him if he was okay.

"You passed out! I don't know what happened. Have you been taking your meds?" asked Shirley.

"How long was I out? I don't even remember falling. And I stopped taking my meds. Maybe that is why I passed out." he responded, puzzled.

"Well, I would suggest you see a doctor if you are passing out like that. Are you going to be okay? It is getting late and I have to get home." She insisted.

"Yes. I will be fine. I am so happy that you stopped by. I had a great time. I will walk you to your car. Please let me know when you get home safely." Said Quincy.

Over the next few weeks, Shirley kept in contact with Quincy. She called every day and dropped by occasionally just to keep tabs on how well he was doing. Then one cold morning, Quincy called Shirley in a panic.

"Hello! Shirley are you there?" said Quincy over the phone. "I don't know what is going on with me. I woke up this morning with this extreme pain around my mouth.

I ran to the bathroom to get a look at myself in the mirror and as soon as I turned on the lights, I saw it.”

“What did you see?” asked Shirley.

“Bumps everywhere! All over my mouth and my face. Sores. I think I have herpes or something. It is horrible, I tell you. But that is not the worst of it.”

“Quincy, what are you talking about? What is not the worst of it? What is going on over there?”

“I took a shower this morning after seeing the herpes. I felt nasty. I felt like I needed to cleanse myself. So I am washing my body, right. I am cleaning my neck, my shoulders, my arms and my chest. All good. And then I get down to my stomach and my pelvic area and that’s when I saw it!”

“Saw what?!! What did you see Quincy?”

“It was the mark of the beast all over my meat. Red and brown rashes everywhere. WTF is happening to me? I just want to die at this point!”

“Don’t say that Quincy! Everything is going to be okay!”

“No it isn’t Shirley!! I will never be the same again. I am tired of all this. HIV and now some other stuff.

I can't live like this. I should have killed myself long ago. I couldn't do it then, but I darn sure can do it now. Yeah. That's what I am going to do! Kill myself"

"NNNOOOO! NO! Don't do that! I am coming right over. Stay where you are and leave the door unlocked." Shirley suggested.

She hung up the phone, called her divine 9 and told them that is was time. They all packed up and hurried to Quincy's. When they got there, Shirley told them to wait outside while she went in. She went up the apartment to the penthouse and opened the door.

"Quincy? You here?" she called as she walked through the rooms of the house. When she got to the master bathroom, she found Quincy sitting on the floor.

"Get up from there. Let's go in the kitchen and talk," she said.

As they made their way to the kitchen, she texted her girls and then sat down at the dining table. As they began to chat, the front door flew open and in came the divine 9 with their equipment.

"Who the hell is that coming through my front door?" Quincy stood up.

"Shut up Quincy and sit your ass down!" Shirley demanded.

"You said that you wanted to die so we are here to put you out of your misery. But first, we've got to humiliate you like you humiliated us. You see Tina over there? Do you remember her? Tina has herpes Quincy. And Suzanne. That college girl that you screwed. She has syphilis. They gave all that to you."

Shirley explained.

"What? Ain't no way. I haven't slept with those two women in years. I tested for Herpes and syphilis years after I was with them so there is no way they gave that to me. LIES!" screamed Quincy!

Ladies, tie his ass up. The ladies grabbed Quincy and tied him to his chair. They used ropes and tape. And then they put a bag over his head.

"I drugged you a few weeks ago. I never knew roofies were for real but they sure did the trick. We had so much fun with your naked body." She and the girls giggled.

"Set up the camera up!"

"If you are going to kill me, kill me now and get it over with!" screamed Quincy.

"Kill you now?! You don't give us orders!" Kesha said.

"We want to show the whole world what happens when they let people like you go free. Why don't you sit there and think of what you'd like to say to the world when you get your ten minutes of fame. And make it good!" said Kesha.

"Good morning America!" said Shirley, as she stood in front of the camera with a microphone.

"I am glad we have your attention. Today, we are going to right what you have wronged. You have freed a guilty man; a killer, a diseased freak that deserves to die, and DIE, HE SHALL! But first, we would like to give him a chance to state his case so that you can hear it for yourselves. He doesn't think he is guilty. He believes we all got HIV on our own. So let's hear what he has to say."

The camera shifted from Shirley to Quincy who was still tied up in a chair with a bag over his head. Tina removed the bag and took off the tape on Quincy's mouth and motioned for him to speak.

"What happened to these women, happened to me too. I got infected with the virus and do you think that person had the decency to tell me? No! She didn't tell me a damn thing nor did she care. I must admit that when I found out that I had this disease, I was upset. I was enraged. But then I realized that what happened to me was my own fault. I was irresponsible. I could have prevented this from happening but I didn't. I didn't wear a condom and I didn't make my partner get tested either. I did what mostly everyone else does; I took a lot of chances thinking it could never happen to me. And it didn't happen to me for a long time. But I was very naive. I am not now.

I know that anyone can get AIDs/HIV at anytime, anywhere. Pretty people can get it. Old people. Yooung people. Even kids and babies can get it.

Blacks, whites and Hispanics; anyone. AIDs doesn't discriminate. It only takes one night of unprotected sexual acts and you can get it. And that's what happened to these women. They took one too many chances and now look at them. A condom could have saved their lives. Even me wearing a condom could have saved them.

But are you really going to make me responsible for their lives? Do you really think that these women could have continuously practiced their sex routines and not run into HIV one day? Believe me, HIV was bound to happen to them sooner or later just as it happened to me.

Don't feel sorry for them America, because I don't. I don't even feel sorry for myself. What happened to them is their fault. They made the choice to have unprotected sex. They were irresponsible and there is no excuse for it. And if you, America, continues the same irresponsible sexual acts, you too will be a victim of this disease. One day someone will do to you what some woman did to me and what I've done to these women.

You have one choice America: Will you choose to protect yourself and prevent diseases from happening? Will you limit the amount of partners you are sleeping with on the regular? Will you and your partner get tested? Or will you continue practicing unprotected sex and blame everyone else for your misfortune like these women?

Whichever choice you make, know that you will be the one responsible for the consequences. What happens, happens because of you. It will be your decision. You are the parent of your life. What you say goes. I know you want me to apologize America, but that's something I just cannot do. I would rather die to prove a point rather than live and take the blame for someone else's mistakes. That's all that I have to say.

And with that said, the camera was turned back to Shirley. "You hear that America? He still thinks he isn't guilty, but we don't care what he thinks. He's still guilty in our book. Look at his face! Look at it!" Shirley screamed.

The camera zoomed in on Quincy's face so that everyone could see his herpes.

"You see that? That's what they call Syphilis. And that?

Herpes! Need I go on? Gonorrhea, Chlamydia, whatever you name, he's got it! Now I am going to set him free so that he can go out and have sex with all your daughters and maybe your sons too and infect them all. And when he is done, I will find him a good lawyer to get him off the hook. Is that what you want me to do America? Let him go? Let him roam the streets infecting people?"

Shirley paused and looked straight into the camera.

"Well, today is your lucky day America, because I am not going to do that. Unlike Quincy, I've got some morals. But I tell you what I am going to do. I'm going to save you some trouble and take this man out of his misery."

Shirley grabbed the knife and walked towards Quincy.

"Wait! Wait! I have one more thing to say." Quincy begged. "You may kill me Shirley, but you and that syphilis chick are going to hell right along with me. After all these years, you still haven't learned your lesson, have you?

I found out 6 months ago that I have stage 3 HIV, FULL BLOWN AIDS BABY!! And you got it too since you couldn't stay away from this penis. Even after the court case, you couldn't stay way. Why are you so desperate for a man? And now, you have AIDs. AIDS, AIDS, AIDS!! You can thank your AIDs donor!" Quincy started laughing hysterically.

Shirley couldn't move. She was at a loss for words. She took a deep breath. Her body started trembling. She dropped the knife and fell to the floor. Then before she could let out a cry, Kesha came over, picked up the knife, walked over to Quincy and cut his throat. The AIDs blood poured. The show was over.